MORE THAN A SURVIVOR

A Story of Hope and Healing

BY

SHERRY A. SIMS

To Donna
From Sheila
9-23-15
We will do this
TOGETHER!!!

16 15 14 13   10 9 8 7 6 5 4 3 2 1

More Than a Survivor
ISBN: 978-1-939570-07-9
Copyright © 2013 by Sherry A. Sims.

The story you are about to read is true. Various names and identifying details have been changed to protect the privacy of individuals. This book details the experiences of the author. It is not meant to be used, nor should it be used, to diagnose or treat a medical condition. For diagnosis or treatment options, consult a physician. The publisher and author are not engaged in rendering medical advice. Should you require medical or other expert assistance, you should seek the services of a competent professional.

Published by Word & Spirit Publishing.
P.O. Box 701403
Tulsa, OK 74170

Cover Design by Paige1Media
Cover Image by Gentry Photography

TABLE OF CONTENTS

CHAPTER I

WHEN YOU LEAST EXPECT IT

Nobody expects a crisis to happen, or a miracle for that matter, especially when you're a 34-year-old newlywed. But when it does, it changes everything. I know. It happened to me.

It was a Wednesday night in June when, after a long day at work, I stepped out of my clothes and into a hot shower. My husband Doug and I were living in an upper middle-income suburb of Dallas then. We had just moved from Oklahoma ten months earlier, right after a whirlwind courtship and marriage. Probably not the best idea I've ever had.

Dallas was fascinating and I loved the fast pace. But I was still adjusting to the new husband, the new job, the new house. The new stepchildren were probably the hardest adjustment. Doug had two boys from a previous marriage and because he still felt guilty about his divorce four years earlier and leaving them to move further away, all of their visits were geared toward fulfilling their every wish. My 15-year-old daughter was also having problems adjusting, which made things even more difficult. It was a tough way to start a marriage. Obviously not the fairy tale beginning I had hoped for.

But I was determined to look on the bright side. I was the director of sales and marketing in the new regional office for a prominent automobile lease finance company. We lived in a beautiful ranch-style brick home. We were getting involved in a local church, and I had already made some great friends. It was the new beginning I needed, and I was going to make it work.

Water ran down my back and shoulders as I washed my hair, enjoying the scented shampoo. After washing the rest of my body, I did something I had never done before—a breast exam.

I first became familiar with self-exams five years earlier. My roommate at the time had an instruction card hanging in the bathroom, so I knew how to do it. But it wasn't until I saw the information featured on a news segment earlier that week that I decided it might be a good habit to start.

So I faced the water and lifted my right arm above my head. Gingerly, I touched around the perimeter of my breast with my left hand. I hadn't gotten far when I stopped. Suddenly, I focused in on what

I was feeling—something small and hard on the side of my right breast. *I must be imagining things.* I pressed more firmly and felt it again. It was like a stone, but perfectly round and about the size of a pea. Something was wrong.

Water continued to run down my face and neck, but I stood there stunned, staring numbly at the place where I had felt the lump. How long had it been there? I quickly examined the other breast. Nothing. Suddenly one word came to mind: Cancer. I felt the lump again. *Oh God, I have cancer! No, I'm jumping to conclusions. It can't be. Could it? It must be something else.* I struggled as dark thoughts tried to overpower me. *NO. It had to be something else. It just had to be. Perhaps this was normal. But if it was normal, wouldn't there be another lump on the other side? But there wasn't.* I was in shock, terrified of the unknown.

After my shower, I found myself staring into the long vanity mirror hanging above my sink. My reflection seemed unfamiliar. Moments before, I was just a regular person. Sure I had problems—stresses—but nothing I couldn't handle. With one chance breast exam everything had changed. But I couldn't let the fear overwhelm me. I had to pull it together. I had to tell Doug.

I crawled into bed next to my husband.

"Doug? Are you still awake?"

"Hmm," he answered.

"Doug, I found something," I whispered. No answer. I turned to face him and took his hand from under the covers. Placing it on my right breast, I said, "I found a lump."

"A lump?" he repeated, half asleep.

I answered, "Yes, can you feel that? I'm not sure what it is."

"It's probably nothing," he said.

"Doug!"

"Look," he said, "if it's still there in a week or so, go to the doctor and have it checked out." And that was it.

A week or so? Really? Obviously this wasn't **his** body we were talking about! I had no idea what was going on, and I wasn't going to wait to find out. I said goodnight, rolled over, and called my gynecologist the next morning.

CHAPTER 2

THE BATTLE BEGINS

Lying flat on my back, I stared at the bright fluorescent lights. The exam room was freezing and the paper gown I was wearing was not helping at all. A month before I had been in the same room, having my annual pelvic exam. At the time Dr. Cline, my gynecologist, gave me three packets of Loestrin, a birth control pill to help balance my hormones. My mood swings were getting out of control and he thought the Loestrin might help. If anyone needed help, I did.

Dr. Cline was a down-to-earth man in his mid-forties with a pleasant smile. After he checked the lump, I asked if I should be concerned.

"How long have you had this?" he asked, checking the other breast.

"I found it two days ago," I said.

"Well then, I wouldn't worry about it," he said, touching the lump one more time. "It's probably just a glandular reaction."

"To what?" I asked.

He took off his green plastic gloves and moved to lean against a small counter on the opposite side of the room.

"The Loestrin," he answered. "Still having mood swings?" By now, he had picked up my chart and was pulling a silver pen from the monogrammed pocket of his shirt.

"Maybe you should ask my husband," I said half-smiling, then sitting up.

He turned, grinning over his shoulder. "You should level off soon. We'll see how you're doing in about a month."

"But, what about this?" I said, pointing to my right breast.

He looked at my file on the counter and scribbled something down. "Whatever it is, it will probably be gone the next time I see you."

Really? That's it? Suddenly, I felt an overwhelming sense of relief. "I'm really glad to hear that," I said, trying to close the chilly gap in the front of the disposable gown. "Can I get dressed now?"

Nodding on the way out of the door, he reminded me to make another appointment with the receptionist.

"Whew, I'm glad that's over," I said, reaching for my clothes.

Unfortunately, I had spoken too soon.

Daily, like a pregnant woman checking the size of her belly, I faithfully checked the lump every time I went to the bathroom. I kept hoping it would disappear, but it didn't. By the next month, the small hard mass had doubled in size. At my next appointment with Dr. Cline, I was worried and more than a little upset.

"Are you sure?" I said when he once again tried to reassure me that everything was fine and that the lump was probably just a glandular reaction to my medication. "Look how big it is!"

Then I voiced the dreaded thought that hadn't left my mind for a month. "What if it's cancer?"

He looked me in the eye. "Sherry, listen. You're only 34 years old. You don't smoke, you have no history of cancer in your family. You don't meet the criteria."

"But it's getting bigger every day," I insisted. "And if it's not cancer, what could it be?"

"We'll draw some blood today and see what we find. Okay?"

"But Doctor—?"

"Listen, Sherry. We'll keep an eye on it. So, don't worry. Breast cancer is not something you need to be concerned with, okay?" He smiled and gently patted my leg.

Reluctantly, I held my peace. But I knew something serious was going on. Medically he knew more than I did, but I was the one with a foreign object growing inside my body!

Over the next few days I continued to monitor the ever-expanding lump. When it had grown to the size of a quarter, I knew it was time to talk to my gynecologist again. Well, the third time was the charm. This time Dr. Cline quickly ordered a mammogram.

Chapter 3

MAMMOGRAMS

Seven days later, I had my first mammogram. On the scale of unpleasant procedures, a mammogram falls somewhere between a pap smear and a root canal. At the time, I didn't realize the "impact" a mammogram would have on me, even though a cartoon taped to the wall of my changing area should have told me something.

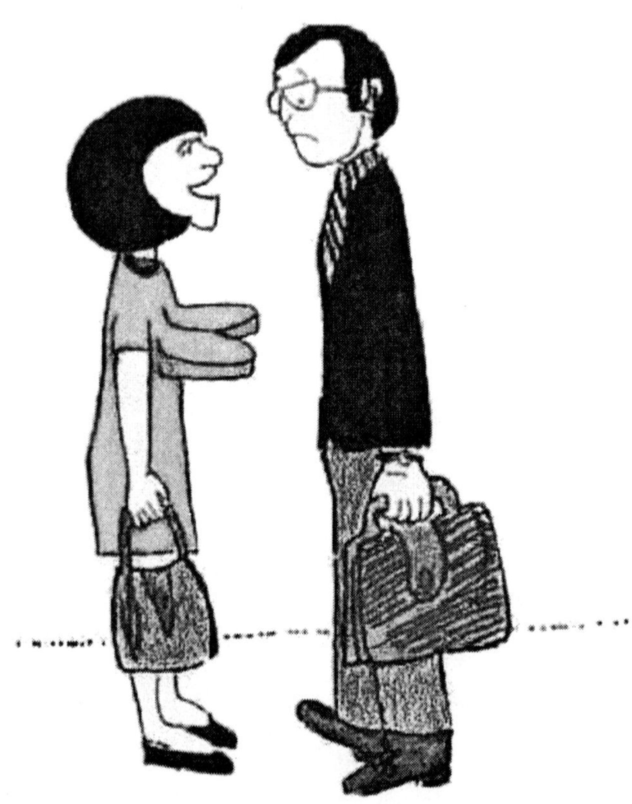
YES, I DID HAVE MY MAMMOGRAM
TODAY... WHY DO YOU ASK?

I'm not sure why it's always cold in medical buildings, but the changing area at the imaging center was no different. I reluctantly took off my clothes, hung them on two metal hooks, and quickly wiped my breasts and underarms with a moistened towelette as instructed. Then picking up the provided garb—another paper gown—I quickly put it on.

"So, how are you today?" the technician asked as she led me across the cold tile.

"Freezing," I said, while crossing my arms to keep the gown closed in front.

"I know," she said gently, "I'm sorry about that. Is this your first mammogram?"

I nodded, eying the machine. It looked like a giant microscope.

"Well, don't worry; we'll get you in and out as quick as we can."

Nodding, I wondered what she meant by that. I soon found out.

Once we started the procedure, I tried hard to concentrate on the constant hum of the machine instead of the awkward poses I had to endure. *Now the cartoon made perfect sense,* I thought. Thankfully, the mammogram didn't take long and I hoped, as I put my clothes back on, it would be a long time until I had to endure another one.

Within 72 hours, Dr. Cline's nurse called to tell me what I had already known; the mammogram showed an unidentified mass in my right breast. Since Dr. Cline didn't have a base-line mammogram to compare these most recent results with, his nurse wanted to know if I would go back in for another mammogram. *Oh, Lord, not again.* But this time, my desperate need to know what the lump was far outweighed my dread of yet another unpleasant experience. My second mammogram took place a week later.

On Wednesday after the second mammogram, another nurse from Dr. Cline's office called with the results. The mysterious lump had been upgraded to a suspicious mass, but the doctor couldn't determine exactly what the mass was without a needle biopsy.

Biopsy?

"Doesn't a biopsy mean it's cancer?" I asked nervously.

"No, it just means we need more information," the nurse said.

"But a biopsy—"

"We'll have the receptionist call you later today with an appointment time. It'll probably be this week."

"It's serious, isn't it?" I said. I felt dizzy again, like I had when I first found the lump in the shower.

"The doctor won't know until after the biopsy," she said curtly. "We'll let you know about your appointment later today."

Numbly, I sat holding the phone to my ear. Somehow it didn't make sense. For two months, the doctor had been telling me nothing was wrong. Now everything was happening so fast and yet they still weren't telling me anything. What did that mean? It couldn't be cancer, could it? I was only 34 years old. Surely it was something else.

I needed some advice. *Oh God, please send someone who can help me understand what's going on...*

CHAPTER 4

A FRAGILE HOPE

After church that night, I made a beeline for the pastor's wife, a strong, beautiful woman I had come to admire during the few short months we had attended their church. Although I didn't know Beverly Earley very well, I felt I could trust her, so I eagerly pulled her aside in the small sanctuary.

"I found a lump several weeks ago," I explained, laying my hand near my right breast, "and now the doctor wants to do a biopsy. I'm not sure what's going on." I felt my face flush slightly. Until then, only Doug and I had known about the situation. Suddenly it felt strange to talk about it—to finally admit it—to someone else.

Beverly looked concerned. "What are they saying? Is it cancer?"

"They don't know yet. I have a needle biopsy scheduled this Friday," I said.

Her husband, Bill, joined us and, at Beverly's request, I filled him in. "Is there anything we can do for you?" he asked. Bill Earley was a kind, compassionate man with a charismatic personality. Standing there, I was grateful for their support and thankful for their church which God led us to just in time.

"I don't know," I said quickly. "I'm not sure what I'm going to do. I just wish someone would tell me what is going on!"

Suddenly Beverly looked away and started scanning the small groups of people scattered around the sanctuary. "Sherry, do you know Anna? Anna Roberts?" she asked. I shook my head no.

"She's on duty tonight," Bill reminded Beverly, and then said to me, "Anna is a registered nurse at Arlington Memorial. I know she'd be glad to answer your questions if she can."

"Really?" I said hopefully. "That would be great!"

"Do you want us to have her call you tomorrow?" Beverly asked.

"Yes, that would be perfect," I said, relieved. Finally. Someone I could talk to who could help me sort things out! I had tried to discuss all of this with Doug, but he didn't say much. Anna sounded like an answer to prayer.

From the time I got home from work on Thursday, I waited anxiously for the phone to ring. It finally did ring, around 6:00 p.m. After our brief introductions, I quickly summarized the whole situation and asked Anna what she thought. "Is it cancer?" I asked.

She was quiet for a moment. "Probably not," she answered. "I mean, you're only 34 years old with no family history of cancer and you don't smoke. Cancer seems pretty unlikely. It's probably just a cyst."

"A cyst? What is that exactly?"

"It's like a bubble with fluid in it."

"So is a cyst considered cancer?" I asked.

"No, cancer is something entirely different. Cysts are usually easy to treat. Actually, if it is a cyst, the surgeon may decide to drain it during the needle biopsy procedure."

"That sounds messy," I said. But it certainly sounded better than cancer!

"Don't worry, Sherry. I'm sure everything will be fine," Anna said before she hung up.

I let out a deep breath and felt myself relax. Surely Anna was right. As a registered nurse, she had probably seen dozens of cases like mine: women who thought they had cancer, but only had cysts. Hopefully, that's what I had—just a cyst.

The truth was, at that point, I needed some good news. So I stubbornly clung to every word Anna had told me. The very thought of the mysterious lump being a drainable cyst and not cancer gave me an enormous amount of comfort. Even though the biopsy was the next day, I slept better that night than I had in months.

Chapter 5

NEEDLE BIOPSY

The needle biopsy wasn't until 3:00 in the afternoon. I left work around 2:30 p.m., even though the surgeon's office was just two miles away. In Dallas, you never knew about the traffic, and I didn't want to be late. I was so ready for all of this health nonsense to be over with so life could get back to normal.

Once in the surgeon's examination room, I met Dr. Frank. With wire-rimmed glasses and a pocket protector, he looked more like a CPA than a doctor. Dr. Frank did not believe in chitchat. After handing me yet another dreaded paper gown, he methodically instructed me to change, and then lie flat on the exam table. Then he left the room. Definitely lacking in bedside manner, I hoped his surgical skills were better than his ability to communicate!

He returned moments later holding a syringe with a needle that looked at least four inches long. Silently, he moved the right half of my gown aside and dabbed the skin over the lump with a local anesthetic. I set my eyes on the white ceiling tiles directly above. After a moment I began to feel a dull pressure.

"What do you do for a living?" Dr. Frank said out of the blue.

"I'm in sales," I answered. I felt the pressure increase. Maybe he was draining the cyst.

"And where do you live?" he asked. All of a sudden, Mr. Stoic wanted to make small talk?

"In the mid-cities area, near Airport Freeway."

"Is it nice there?" he asked. *What was he talking about?*

"Do you mean my neighborhood?" I asked, turning to look at him. His brow was wrinkled with concern. I followed his eyes to the syringe and the ugly, dark fluid he was extracting from the lump.

"Yes," I said, moving my eyes back toward the ceiling. Anna had said the fluid would probably be clear. *Don't panic,* I told myself, *maybe it's a different kind of cyst.*

"Any children?" he asked.

"Yes. Three," I said, not wanting to explain our blended family.

I felt the pressure suddenly stop. "You can put your clothes back on. Please come by my office before you leave." And just like that, it was over.

Needless to say, being asked by a surgeon to stop by his office to talk felt a lot like being summoned to the principal's office in grade school. Not a pleasant experience. But since I needed to get back to work as soon as possible, I quickly finished dressing and went down the hall to meet him.

Entering the surgeon's office, I reluctantly sat down in a leather chair across from his file-strewn desk. The concern on Dr. Frank's face quickly caused my self-confidence to fade.

"Sherry, the fluid I extracted did not look good," he said. "So, I've decided to schedule you for a surgical biopsy Monday morning at Arlington Memorial."

"But I thought it was just a cyst," I said.

Dr. Frank responded abruptly, "No, it's definitely not a cyst. I'm sending the biopsy to the pathology lab right now. And since I need to know what I'll be dealing with Monday morning, I've put a rush on the reports. You need to go to the hospital immediately for pre-op."

What? I was in shock.

Innocently, I asked what pre-op meant. He quickly explained, "You'll have to fill out some paper-work at the hospital before your surgery and they may have to run a few tests."

"But do I have to do it today? I really need to get—"

"You can't wait. You need to take care of this right now," Dr. Frank said.

Leaving his office in a daze and heading for my car, I realized how concerned the doctor had been. His insistence on moving the process along so quickly brought my original fears to the forefront, kicking and screaming. This was something serious, some-thing that was quickly getting out of control.

It was like being on an emotional see-saw. Every new test result or prognosis either sent me soaring upwards or dropping downwards. As I stood in the parking lot by my car door, I realized I had to make a decision. If I was going to make it through this, I had to keep my emotions level. I had to focus on the important things—pursuing my career and enjoying my family—and let the rest take care of itself. Besides, he hadn't said it was cancer, had he? And maybe over the weekend, things would improve. Maybe the lab results would show that a surgical biopsy wasn't necessary after all. Or maybe, if I still had to have the surgical biopsy, I'd find out the lump wasn't cancer. Maybe it would turn out to be something else. It's amazing what we tell ourselves.

By the time I arrived home from the hospital, it was late and I was exhausted. The pre-op had included several tests, a chest x-ray, and a huge stack of hospital documents to sign. Even though we had the boys for the summer, I was eager to get home. I really needed a reprieve from the emotional battle I was fighting.

On the way home, I realized I hadn't told my parents what I'd been going through. I'd been putting it off, knowing the news would come as a shock, but I knew they believed in miracles and boy, did I need one.

Of course this wasn't the first time I had to call my parents with troubling news. Over the years I had experienced more than my fair share of disappointments, tragedies, and heartbreaks. However, this would be the first time I would call them about a potentially life-threatening disease.

First I talked with Mom, then Dad. They were surprised by the news, but they didn't seem devastated. At least I didn't hear it in their voices. They did get quiet, however, when I first mentioned the lump. They asked all the right questions and let me explain things to the best of my ability. At the end of our conversation, Dad asked if he could pray for me and I quickly said yes. As Dad began to pray, I could hear Mom praying quietly in the background. I felt peaceful.

After promising to call with the biopsy results on Monday, we said our goodbyes. I was so grateful to have parents who supported and encouraged me with their faith instead of fueling my worry with their fear. I wasn't sure if it was their prayers or just talking to them, but after the phone call, I began to feel much better.

CHAPTER 6

THE PHONE CALL

Since the rather lengthy pre-op appointment kept me from getting back to work on Friday, I decided to go in to the office Saturday morning. I knew my desk would be covered with paperwork. Mail and reports and messages were like rabbits. They seemed to multiply like crazy every time I stepped away from my desk.

I decided to take my daughter Stefanie with me. My boss had hired Stefanie to clean the office once a week and having a job seemed to change her. Her outlook became more positive and she was actually becoming more responsible. A paycheck can do that for a teenager.

After giving Stef her instructions and cleaning supplies, I began to tackle my overflowing in-basket. I hadn't been at it that long when the phone rang. Odd. The office was closed on Saturday, but I decided to answer the phone anyway.

"Sherry, is that you? This is Dr. Frank."

Dr. Frank? The surgeon?

"Yes, Dr. Frank," I said.

"Your husband said you were at work," he said, "but I really need to talk to you. Are you sitting down?"

My heart jumped.

"I am now," I said, settling in my chair, holding my breath.

"The lab results came back this morning and it's cancer. So instead of proceeding with the surgical biopsy on Monday, I'd like to do a mastectomy."

I was shocked. "What?" I blurted out. "You've got to be kidding!"

He briefly paused. "No, I'm not kidding," was his curt reply. "Based on your lab results, you need a mastectomy immediately."

I couldn't believe what I was hearing. I was numb.

"Sherry, are you there?" Dr. Frank asked.

"Yes. I'm just surprised," I replied. "Did you say that you want to do a mastectomy on Monday?

"Yes," he answered firmly.

How could I agree to this? I had finally accepted that the mass wasn't a cyst and that I needed a surgical biopsy. Now he's decided to skip the surgical biopsy and wants me to agree to a mastectomy instead? It was just too much.

"No, I don't think so," I said finally.

Now it was Dr. Frank's turn to be surprised. "What do you mean, you don't think so? Why?" he demanded.

I shifted in my seat. "I want to have the biopsy first, like we planned."

"Sherry, this is very serious—" he began.

"I understand. That's why I need to speak with my husband first," I said firmly. There were other reasons I was opting for the biopsy first, but I wasn't prepared to share them with Dr. Frank right then.

Dr. Frank seemed to be put out by the fact I had a mind of my own. He strongly recommended that I reconsider, but when I wouldn't budge, he gave me his home number and told me to call after I talked to Doug. I thanked him and hung up the phone.

As I sat at my desk that Saturday, I felt my emotional see-saw fall. Now it was official. I had *breast cancer.* For months I believed that if I didn't verbalize my fear, then it wouldn't be real. But it was real, and now I had to face it.

"Mom?" Stefanie said. She was standing at the door of my office, her voice trembling. "Are you okay?"

I sat up straight and smiled. "Sure. Why?"

"Who were you talking to?" Stefanie asked. She had overheard my side of the conversation with Dr. Frank.

For two months I hadn't told her anything. I didn't want her to worry. But I knew it was time to come clean. Sort of. "That was just a doctor I went to see yesterday. I found a lump a couple of months ago and we've been trying to figure out what it is."

Stefanie came closer. "A couple of months ago? Why didn't you tell me?"

"Well, I didn't know what to tell you since I didn't know what it was exactly," I said, smiling. "It's no big deal, really."

"Really? So what did the doctor tell you?" Stefanie said, crossing her arms.

I shuffled some papers, still smiling, though it was harder now. "He thinks it's cancer, but don't worry. He said he can take care of it. Are you finished with Larry's office yet?"

She uncrossed her arms. "No. I still have to dust and vacuum."

"Well get with it. You don't want to be here all day, do you?" I said shooing her with one hand and trying to focus on the blur before me.

"No," she said smiling and left the room. When I knew she was far enough away, I started to cry.

Then I called Doug.

That night we took the three kids to a nearby mall to see *Forrest Gump*. The movie had received a lot of positive reviews, so we thought it would be a good choice for the family. Anything would have worked at that point. I just needed a diversion; something to get my mind off the cancer.

Doug and I had hardly talked all night. When I called him from the office and told him what Dr. Frank had recommended, he sided with the doctor. "Well, if that's what needs to happen," Doug said, "then just do it." When I disagreed saying it wasn't a simple decision, he said I was just being difficult!

How could he totally overlook that this was my body we were talking about, not his? I was furious. Did he not understand that if I agreed, I would be the one having my breast amputated! Not only that, but our insurance wouldn't cover an operation at Arlington Memorial. This decision had the potential to add more to the enormous mountain of debt we already had. I was not going to let Doug or the surgeon push me into making a decision I was not ready to make.

So sitting in the theatre, I let the plot of the movie distract me from reality. At least it did until Forrest's mother, played by Sally Field, died of cancer. Needless to say, that ruined the rest of the movie for me.

CHAPTER 7

SECONDS

Just when you think things can't get any worse, they can. Monday morning's biopsy confirmed the cancer was malignant and the breast would have to be removed. Because our insurance required a second opinion from one of their doctors, they gave me the name of Dr. Pauline Stephens, a surgeon who specialized in breast cancer. I contacted her office on Tuesday and scheduled an appointment for the following day.

That night while lying in bed, I felt around the perimeter of each breast. Breast self-exams had become a regular habit of mine. My finger surveyed the now familiar lump on the right. But then I found something on the left, pea-sized and hard as a rock. A lump. It felt exactly like the other one had. No way. Really? Another one?

I needed to pray. I had already prayed many times over the past two months, but this time was different. I was angry. Now there were two lumps to deal with! I turned to my husband.

"Doug, would you pray for me?" Obliging my request, he quietly said a very simple prayer. Then it was my turn.

You see, I was raised in a church where we believed God not only heard our prayers, but He gave us power to stand against anything that tried to hurt us. Now something evil was obviously trying to infiltrate my body and steal my health, and I wasn't going to allow it to continue. No one else had authority over my life; not my surgeon or my husband. Ultimately, the decision to not let the cancer take over my body was up to me, and I had put it off long enough. I wasn't going to take it anymore. It had to end. I balled up my fist and prayed through tears, reminding myself what God promised me in the Bible, and then I demanded the cancer to stop!

Suddenly a deep peace came over me. My worries began to fade. No matter what happened next, somehow I knew everything would be all right because God loved me and wanted the best for me. My future was in His capable hands.

Doug went with me to Dr. Stephens' office the next day for the second opinion. After changing into yet another paper gown, Doug and I sat for what seemed like an eternity in a small examination room, me on the table and he in the only chair. While we waited, I felt for the second lump. It was still there. But the peace from my prayer the night before was still there too, deep beneath the surface. I was glad I was getting a second opinion. At least Dr. Stephens was a woman and would hopefully prove to be more sensitive to my situation than Dr. Frank.

Finally Dr. Stephens walked in. She was very professional looking with short, medium brown hair and glasses. She had a warm smile.

"Good morning, Sherry. I'm Dr. Stephens," she said, reaching for my hand. I shook her hand gratefully. Then she shook Doug's.

"Well, I looked over Dr. Frank's notes, and everything seems to be in order. I'd just like to look for myself if you don't mind."

"Why not?" I said, laying down and exposing my breasts. "Everybody else has!"

Dr. Stephens laughed. "Comes with the territory."

"I guess so," I said with mock sarcasm. It was nice to find a doctor with a sense of humor for a change.

She gently felt the lump on my right breast, perhaps noting the texture and size.

"I found another one last night," I said.

Quickly her bright facial expression faded into concern. "A second one?"

"Here," I pointed below my left breast. She felt the lump.

"It's pretty small," she said, and felt in a wider circle around the area.

I looked at her. "It feels just like the other one did when I first found it."

She finished the exam quickly.

"Get dressed and come see me in my office," she said. Noticing my response to her abruptness, she covered my hand with hers. "Don't worry. I'm sure everything's going to be fine. We just need to talk about it," she said.

While sitting across the desk from Dr. Stephens, my husband and I listened intently. The opinion she gave was not what I had hoped for. She agreed with Dr. Frank that I needed a mastectomy as soon as possible. She also recommended a biopsy on the lump in the left breast at the same time. If the biopsy proved the lump was cancerous, she recommended I have a double mastectomy.

As if that wasn't enough, she dropped another bomb. Since the first lump had grown so rapidly and a second lump had been detected, Dr. Stephens believed it was entirely possible that the cancer had metastasized to the brain, bones, or lungs. That meant *after* the double mastectomy, four months of chemotherapy and/or radiation would be required. I balked. I could not lose both breasts *and* all my hair!

"First, there's no way I'm agreeing to chemotherapy," I blurted.

My husband looked shocked. "Sherry, you have to! If you don't, you could die!"

"I don't care," I insisted. "I'm not going to lose my hair!"

"This is something we can discuss later. Do you have any other questions?" Dr. Stephens said.

"Yes. What about reconstructive surgery?" I asked. "Dr. Frank said I'd have to wait a year, but I'm not going to live a year without breasts. I mean, I may not have much, but I'm pretty partial to what I do have!"

Doug was starting to turn pink.

Dr. Stephens laughed. "Don't worry. I usually recommend reconstructive surgery, and it can be done during the mastectomy. I have a colleague, Dr. Kendall, who does great work. Would you like me to schedule you a personal consultation with him?"

I was shocked. I fully expected her to agree with Dr. Frank like she had on everything else. Finally, some good news! "Yes, please!" I said eagerly and before we left the office, I had an appointment to see Dr. Kendall the next day.

THE BRIGHT LIE

All my life I'd felt bosom-challenged. Unlike most women I knew, my breasts had never fully blossomed. I must have stopped at the budding stage. So the idea of reconstructive surgery was starting to *enhance* the whole mastectomy idea (pun intended). I knew the circumstances weren't ideal, but at least I'd finally get the breast augmentation I'd always wanted. When we walked into Dr. Kendall's office that afternoon, I actually felt giddy.

However, not everyone in the office that day shared my enthusiasm. Sitting there with Doug, I observed women flipping through magazines or talking softly to friends or family members. Every face in the waiting room was so serious. I wondered how many of them had just found out they had breast cancer. Quite a few, I imagined, from the number of hopeless faces I saw.

I then remembered my mom. When I was a child and something would be difficult, she taught me to accept the things I couldn't change and change the things I could. *Make lemonade out of lemons*, she used to say. And that's what I was doing. It was much easier to be cheerful about a breast augmentation than it was a possible double mastectomy.

Diffusing a negative situation with a positive attitude had its benefits. It felt like I had risen above the sadness everyone in the room was dealing with. But I didn't want to be insensitive to their pain, so instead of chatting with Doug about how this visit to the plastic surgeon was like a dream come true, I kept quiet. To talk about such an outlook seemed too much like gloating.

A nurse stepped into the waiting room and barked my name. She was in her late 50s and very serious looking. I knew any attempt at humor with her would be futile. Doug and I obediently followed her into an examination room where she asked me a barrage of questions and then handed me yet another paper gown. With one hand on the doorknob and the other clutching my medical file, she announced the doctor would be there soon. With that, she left.

After changing into the gown, I jumped up on the cold examining table to wait and wait and wait some more. I've never understood why patients are required to be on time for appointments only to wait for hours. It doesn't seem fair. Patients are busy people too and should be given the same courtesy they give their doctor. Besides, patients pay the doctors, not the other way around, right? Shouldn't that be enough motivation for doctors to stay on schedule? But I digress.

Finally the door opened and in stepped a tall, handsome blonde with chiseled features and a bronze tan. The only way I could tell he was a doctor was the lab coat he had on. It was definitely worth the wait. Extending his hand, he introduced himself and then shook hands with my husband.

I barely noticed the same militant nurse standing behind him. She handed Dr. Kendall my chart and then stood at attention by his side.

"Sherry, did you decide on the TRAM flap procedure?" Dr. Kendall asked after giving us some information. We had just viewed a DVD that described the TRAM flap procedure and ended with images of a bikini-clad model running along a white sandy beach after surgery. All I wanted was to look like her.

I nodded yes.

"That would require using your stomach muscle to reconstruct your breast, so let's take a look." I stood up before him and opened my gown, feeling more than a little self-conscious.

"Hmm," he said. "Not a lot of muscle to work with, or fat for that matter."

"Well, if you need more fat, maybe you can do something with this!" I said, turning around and presenting my rather ample bare bottom for inspection. I waited for some reaction at least from the nurse, but she was as stoic as ever.

"I can take care of that too, if you'd like," the doctor said nonchalantly. He must have thought I wanted liposuction. I couldn't help but laugh.

By now my husband's face was a deep shade of red. He quickly gave me "the look" and I calmed down.

"Well, okay then," Dr. Kendall said, quickly flipping through the chart. "We will see you on

Tuesday." He shook our hands again on the way out as his dutiful nurse fell in behind him. On her way out, she abruptly turned and looked at me.

"Also, don't forget to bring a cotton sports-type bra that hooks in the front," she said quickly. "You will need to wear it home from the hospital."

I couldn't help myself. "What size should I bring?" I said with a smile.

"The size you wear, of course," she snorted and marched through the door, firmly closing it behind her.

A big grin spread across my face as I began dressing. Suddenly, Doug jumped up. "Sherry, if you don't stop cracking jokes, they're going to throw us out of here!"

"It's okay," I said. "We were leaving anyway."

CHAPTER 9

AN ANSWER TO PRAYER?

In spite of my impending mastectomy, I entered the church sanctuary Sunday morning bubbling and happy. The reconstruction surgery appeared, to me, to be an "answer to prayer." The mastectomy seemed only like the situation God was using to bring the desired reconstruction about. I knew God hadn't caused the cancer, but it seemed He was using it to give me the desire of my heart.

However, that Sunday I learned something extremely important about God. He thinks a lot differently than I do, and it was my friends, Lisa and Kelly, who taught me that lesson after church.

At the end of the service, Lisa and Kelly motioned frantically for me to stay where I was, as they made their way towards me from the other side of the sanctuary. Those two were quite a pair. Kelly was reserved and petite with auburn hair, while Lisa was taller, blonde, and more animated. Finally they made it through the congregation and greeted me with warm hugs and a variety of questions.

"Sherry, you look great. How are you doing?" inquired Kelly.

"Is your surgery still scheduled for Tuesday morning?" Lisa asked.

"Yes, it is!" I said excitedly.

They both looked shocked at my enthusiasm.

"And you're excited?" Lisa asked, her eyebrows raised.

"Well, yes, sort of. Actually, I went to see the plastic surgeon on Thursday and he said he could do the breast reconstruction at the same time as the mastectomy. Isn't that great? You see, I've always needed a little help in that department, if you know what I mean. So this could be a real answer to prayer."

"That's grea—" Kelly started.

"An answer to whose prayer?" Lisa asked. "I've been praying for you to be healed. And you are looking at this as an opportunity to increase your bust size? What are you thinking?"

It was as if Lisa had thrown a bucket of cold water in my face. What was I thinking? Had I been so deceived that I now believed having breast cancer was an answer to prayer? How warped and twisted! In my effort to make something positive out of such a negative situation, I had justified a lie!

"Wow. You're right, I—"

With one hand Lisa grabbed my left hand and with the other hand she grabbed Kelly's right. She then prayed that the cancer would disintegrate and leave my body completely. Afterward Lisa hugged me and promised to come by the hospital on Tuesday.

While discussing my plans after surgery, Kelly and I made our way to the church entrance. We had just walked outside onto the front steps of the church, which faced a busy intersection, when Kelly quickly turned toward me.

"Sherry, doesn't the Bible say we can lay hands on the sick and they will recover?"

"Sure, it does," I nodded.

She then proceeded, "Would you mind if I laid hands on you and prayed?"

"Of course not," I said, thinking one more prayer couldn't hurt.

So there I was, facing a busy street full of cars when Kelly stepped in front of me, placed both her hands on my breasts, and began to pray! If she hadn't been so sincere, I would have died of embarrassment. Instead, I couldn't help but smile as I listened to the words she spoke with such childlike faith. What could have been one of my most embarrassing moments quickly turned into one of my most humbling experiences.

I wonder how God is going to answer those prayers, I thought as we drove home from church. It didn't take long to find out.

//Chapter 10

SURGERY

Blush—check! Lipstick—check! Finally I finished applying my makeup and smiled. The hospital's pre-op instructions prohibited makeup, but there was no way I was going under the knife without my face on. Seriously? Did they really expect me to come out of surgery looking like death warmed over? I don't think so! I was going to go through this operation with as much dignity as possible.

Looking in the mirror one last time, I noticed how calm I seemed and wondered why. Maybe it was because I felt more secure now that my parents had arrived from Oklahoma. Or maybe it was because my pastor and his wife promised to come to the hospital and pray with me again before surgery. Or perhaps it was the get-well card I received from Doug's ex-wife—she had written such a kind note. That was totally unexpected. Regardless of the reason, I felt an overwhelming sense of peace going into surgery that day. Somehow, I knew everything would be all right.

It was getting late and I needed to get to the hospital. Even though my surgery was scheduled for 10:30 a.m., I had to be there no later than 8:30 a.m. This was one appointment I knew I couldn't be late for.

Once we arrived at the hospital, everything switched into overdrive and a whirlwind of activity enveloped me. The next thing I knew, I was situated on a gurney and headed down a long hall toward surgery. But right before I slipped through the double doors into the operating room, I heard voices yelling for us to stop. It was my pastor and his wife running to catch up with me. The orderly abruptly brought the gurney to a screeching halt.

Bill and Beverly began to pray, asking for God's hand to be upon the surgical team, the nurses, the anesthesiologists, and all who had a part to play in the surgical procedure. They prayed the surgery would go smoothly, that there would be no complications, and that the results would be better than expected and that I would experience a swift and miraculous recovery.

"Sherry," Beverly said, "don't worry about a thing. God has everything under control."

I nodded and smiled and the next thing I knew, I was traveling quickly through two sets of double doors into a brightly lit, sterile environment. I felt myself being lifted off the gurney and placed on a cold surgical table. While covering me with layers of warm blankets, the nurses complimented my makeup. I couldn't help but smile.

The only thing I remember after that was the anesthesiologist asking me to count backwards from 100. I got as far as 98. The next thing I heard was a distant voice coaxing me back to consciousness.

"Sherry? Sherry? Are you awake? Surgery's over. Everything went great! How are you feeling? You still have your lipstick on! Amazing! We're going to take you to recovery for a little while and when you're ready, we'll take you to your room, okay?"

CHAPTER 11

A MIRACLE

My time in recovery was a blur. What I do remember was a tall male nurse wheeling me down a long hallway past other patients' rooms. I heard a lot of laughing and loud voices. After being under heavy anesthetic for almost six hours, the noise seemed almost deafening. *Don't they know this is a hospital full of sick people?*

Suddenly my gurney slowed and came to a stop. "Room 1287," the male nurse said. "This is you."

Ironically, all the talking and laughing I heard was coming from my room where at least twelve exuberant people were crowded around an empty hospital bed. Like the Red Sea, the crowd quickly parted to let my gurney through.

After helping me into my hospital bed and rearranging my IVs, the male nurse reluctantly left me in the midst of the rambunctious crowd. Their enthusiasm was almost overwhelming—not to mention a bit confusing. Everyone seemed so light-hearted and not the least bit concerned about my condition. *Why were they all so happy? Didn't they know I had just been through a major operation?*

Bewildered and still feeling the effects of the anesthetic, I spotted my mother, who was standing near the bed. "Mom, what's going on?" I asked.

"Don't you know?" she replied.

"Know what?" I answered.

She leaned in toward my face and smiled. "They didn't find anything!"

"Didn't find anything?" I said in disbelief. "What do you mean, they didn't find anything?"

Anxious to give me the details, she pulled up a chair and sat down. The room got quiet. "When the surgical team did the mastectomy procedure on the right side, all they found in the breast tissue were fragments of the cancer that had disintegrated."

"What?"

"Then, when they biopsied the second lump, they determined it was just fatty tissue."

"What?!" I said again, my voice an octave higher.

"Then," she said, putting her hand on my arm, "when they tested all twenty-six lymph nodes for cancer, they all came back negative! They didn't find anything!"

As she finished, the crowd erupted with excitement. An older gentleman from our church, standing at the foot of my bed, spoke up. "Sixteen years ago, my wife was healed of breast cancer and she's still cancer-free! What God did for her, Sherry, He's done for you. It's a miracle!"

It was slowly sinking in. The surgical team had been prepared to do a double mastectomy and expected to find cancer in all my lymph nodes, yet they didn't find anything. *Had I really received a miracle?*

I had heard stories of others who had experienced supernatural interventions like this. I knew miracles happened. But this was me—imperfect me. No one knew more than I how unworthy I was. But miracles happen because God loves us in spite of us. How humbling to think that God loved *me* enough to change the molecular structure in my body or to send an immune booster to completely obliterate the cancer. Somehow, He had changed everything, present and future, in just a few short hours. I was so grateful.

Then a new thought began to develop. Perhaps this miracle wasn't just about me. *What if my life had been spared for a reason?* But what was it? Obviously, God was the only one who knew *why* He chose to heal me the way He did. Maybe there was a purpose. And if so, I was determined to find out what it was.

Chapter 12

OTHER BATTLES TO WIN

The following day I was propped up in the hospital bed visiting with my parents when Dr. Stephens stopped by. She looked a little bewildered. "Well Sherry," she said, "I guess everything's all right."

"Yes, I guess everything is," I answered with a smile.

Dr. Stephens looked even more uncomfortable when my father began to comment on the miracle I had received. Although she respectfully acknowledged his statement with a smile, she offered no sign of agreement. I guess I couldn't expect her to. When my father finished, she turned to me again.

"By the way, Sherry, I've asked the oncologist to come by and talk with you about treatment options."

My smile quickly disappeared. *She must be joking. Treatment options?*

"But I thought you didn't find anything?" I asked.

"We didn't," she said bluntly. "But I think it would be a good idea if you talked with Dr. Bennett anyway. I asked him to stop by to see you today."

Without giving me a chance to reply, Dr. Stephens turned, shook hands with both of my parents, waved goodbye to me, and quickly left the room. I couldn't believe it. Not only did she not acknowledge the miracle, but she was sending an oncologist to discuss cancer treatment options, even though I had been opposed to treatment before my surgery!

Later that afternoon, Dr. Bennett stopped by. He was shorter than I expected, around 5' 6," and balding with a fair complexion. If he had not introduced himself, I would never have guessed he was an oncologist. He motioned to the chair next to my bed and asked if he could sit down and chat with me for a few minutes. I felt like telling him to save his breath, but instead, I was determined to be nice and reluctantly agreed.

"Sherry," he began quietly, "I talked with Dr. Stephens and, considering the type of breast cancer you were diagnosed with, I would recommend you undergo chemotherapy treatment for the next six months."

Suddenly, my mouth dropped open. "Excuse me? Did you say *six* months?" He nodded sheepishly.

Surely he was mistaken because even before surgery, when Dr. Stephens suspected the cancer had metastasized, she only recommended four months of treatment. Surely he had not heard the good news!

"Doctor," I said as evenly as I could, "can you tell me why you're recommending six months of chemotherapy when they didn't find anything during my surgery yesterday?"

He explained. "Well, six months of chemotherapy is our standard recommendation for this type of breast cancer. It—"

"But why, Doctor, should I even consider treatment when they didn't find anything?"

"Good question," he said as if he'd never heard such a question before, which was a little scary. Didn't anyone question oncologists about their proposed treatment plans? Or did patients just blindly obey, subjecting their bodies to whatever was suggested? By now I knew hair loss was minor compared to some of chemotherapy's other side effects. Radiation could be even worse. Chemotherapy was like a war between poisons—chemo and cancer—only it was the rest of the person's body that was often the biggest casualty.

"You'd be receiving chemotherapy as a preventative measure," he said. "This type of breast cancer is extremely aggressive and there is a good chance it may reoccur if—"

"Dr. Bennett," I said with a forced grin, "*if* I agreed to the six months of chemotherapy you recommend, can you guarantee I will never have breast cancer again?"

I could see the wheels turning as he looked through my medical file positioned on his lap. A few seconds later he said, "Well, considering you're still very young, and you're not a smoker or a heavy drinker and you have no history of breast cancer in your family, I believe after you undergo six months of chemotherapy I could guarantee you a 33 percent chance of never having breast cancer again."

I had to stifle a laugh. "Thirty-three percent? Really? That's all?"

"Sherry, any chance—"

"Dr. Bennett, if you don't mind, I think I'll pass."

Realizing my mind was made up, he handed me a couple of oncology brochures and left. Just like that, the conversation was over. No chemotherapy.

My hospital room filled with silence as I leaned back on my pillow. At first I had refused the chemo because I didn't want to lose my hair. But it was the miracle that gave me the confidence to refuse it this time. I couldn't believe it. Just a few short days ago there had been cancer in my body, and now it was gone. Once again I wondered why.

That second day in the hospital drifted into the next. I began to lose track of time. Before I knew it, three days had passed and I was anxious to go home.

That morning, one of the plastic surgeons from the surgical team stopped by to check on me. Dr. Graham was his name—a kind man, and boisterous. After looking over my chart, he mentioned that Dr. Stephens had ordered a bone scan.

I felt my heart suddenly fall. A bone scan? Why? Did Dr. Stephens know something she wasn't telling me, or was she just trying to disprove the miracle? Before the surgery, she had predicted the cancer might have metastasized to the brain, bones, or lung. Maybe this was her final attempt to locate the cancer that had miraculously disappeared. Either way, it wasn't long before I heard the gurney wheels clanking down the hall toward my room. Well, I guess now I could add a bone scan to my growing list of new experiences.

Although the scan was entirely painless, fear started to grip me as the cold realization set in. *What if Dr. Stephens was right? What if the cancer had metastasized to the bones? What would I do then? What if…?*

I realized I had to get a grip on my emotions. I couldn't let fear take over! After returning to my room, I asked Mom to give me the box of books and cassette tapes she had brought from home. I needed something to distract me from my negative thoughts. As I rummaged through the box, I ran across a cassette tape by a minister named Jerry Savelle called *You've Come Too Far to Quit!* That was it. Exactly what I needed. There was no way I could give up now. I was determined.

Listening to that little cassette tape not only helped me pass the time, but its words of encouragement began to calm the debilitating fear and anxiety I felt. My attitude started to change. I knew with certainty that I had come too far to quit! In my heart, I knew everything would be all right. Why wouldn't it be? Everything else had worked out. Why wouldn't this? I had to have FAITH! I couldn't just HOPE, I had to BELIEVE things were going to be okay and somehow, I knew they would!

Just as the tape ended and the cassette player clicked off, the door to my room swung open and Dr. Graham walked in, smiling.

"Well, Sherry, are you ready to go home?" he asked.

"Absolutely, but what about the results from the bone scan?"

"Didn't they tell you?" he said. "It was all clear, no problem. Let's get you out of here, so you can enjoy the rest of the weekend."

Again I was amazed, not just about the bone scan results, but I was being released after only three days in the hospital. Originally I was told it would be at least a week before I would go home. Everything was not just all right; it was even better than I could have hoped.

"Oh, by the way," Dr. Graham said, "since you're going home earlier than expected, would you mind coming by my office on Sunday? I have to remove the staples from your incisions within five days or they'll leave a scar."

"About what time and how long will it take?" I asked. "I'm going to church on Sunday."

Almost laughing, he replied, "You might be getting ahead of yourself a little. I don't think you're going to feel much like going to church so soon after surgery."

Half grinning I replied, "Oh, I'm going. Once I make up my mind, nothing can change it. And besides, how could I NOT go to church after all that's happened?"

Shaking his head in disbelief, Dr. Graham's smile grew bigger. "It will take about 15 minutes. Can you be at my office by 8:00 a.m.?"

"I'll be there!" I said, feeling at least ten feet tall.

CHAPTER 13

MORE GOOD NEWS

Thirty-six hours later, I was slowly putting on a pair of black pantyhose, trying not to dislodge the two drainage tubes still protruding from my TRAM flap incisions. All that was left were my dress and shoes, and I'd be ready to go. I promised Dr. Graham I'd be at his office by 8:00 a.m., and so far everything was right on schedule. I love proving people wrong, especially when they tell me I can't do something. Soon all the discomfort I was experiencing would be forgotten when I saw the look on his face.

Doug drove me up to the main entrance of the hospital and suggested I use a wheelchair, but I said no. Determined to walk in unassisted, I pushed open the passenger door. Deliberately placing my feet on the ground, I stood up and baby-stepped my way through the double doors. I was quite a sight, I'm sure!

Dr. Graham and his two nurses were standing behind the Information Desk in the atrium with their mouths hanging open in surprise. "I can't believe it," smiled the plastic surgeon. "Before you got here, we were wagering as to whether you would actually show up dressed for church or not. I guess we were all wrong!" he added.

Once upstairs in the examination room, Dr. Graham quickly removed the surgical staples from the mastectomy and stomach incisions. Although I had been told before I left the hospital that the remaining two drains would not be removed for another week, he took those out as well.

"Sherry, not only was the outcome of your surgery fantastic, but your recovery has been remarkable," Dr. Graham said. "Your surgery took hours less than expected, you were released from the hospital in half the allotted time, and your incisions are healing twice as fast too! It's just amazing!"

When he finished his work, he announced, "Well, you're all set. Hope I didn't make you late for church." With a wink and a smile he added, "Now I understand why you've been so determined to go."

He had no idea.

Even though we were a few minutes late for the service, I knew our timing was perfect when we opened the sanctuary doors and heard the congregation singing a familiar song. *Look what the*

Lord has done, He healed my body. He touched my mind. He saved me just in time.

I felt the sweet presence of God surround me, filling me with hope. Not only had I survived one of the most feared diseases on the planet, but I was still strong and healthy, still moving forward. With God's help, I had faced a giant and won. The cancer chapter of my life was finally closed. I had a feeling a new chapter was just beginning.

CHAPTER 14

FROM CANCER TO CALL

In the months and years that followed my miracle, I realized God expected me to do my part to remain cancer free. My body was His gift to me and He expected me to take care of it, so I did. Instead of being lax about my health, I became fanatical. Extreme. Every bite of food was carefully scrutinized. Was it healthy enough? Organic? How about antioxidants? And I began to exercise daily, not to look good, but to keep my body and immune system healthy and strong. When hormonal imbalances increased, I sought out homeopathic remedies and avoided synthetic drugs like they were the plague.

Eventually I became less fanatical and more pragmatic, and it was somewhere during that time that God showed me why I was spared—why I had escaped relatively unharmed from such a devastating disease.

You see, the more people I talk to, the more I realize the horrors of cancer and all the damage and pain it often leaves in its wake. I realize the scope of its physical toll on bodies and its emotional toll on marriages (even my own, which ended in divorce). I realize that even those who survive the cancer, chemotherapy, and radiation deal with physical, emotional, and financial scars long after lumps are removed. People often become life-long victims. Instead of moving forward, many sit very still, like a stalked deer, waiting for the annual checkup that will confirm their worst fears—that the cancer has returned. Then they begin the struggle all over again, hoping they can outlast the killer disease a second or third time. Meanwhile they watch timidly, helplessly, as their lives pass them by.

No, my miracle isn't just about me being healed. It is about me encouraging others to not just survive cancer, but to rise to the occasion and conquer it. I want to empower others and inspire them with my faith, letting them know they have the power to not just survive, but to surmount! No, not every person with cancer will receive a miracle, but they can certainly become educated and motivated to prevent and fight cancer. I believe my life was spared for those who need to be encouraged to keep fighting and to keep believing.

Are you someone who needs to be encouraged? Remember this. Regardless of what doctors, family, or even you believe about the situation, don't give up. Fight! If someone came to your house and tried to rob you of your children, your car, or your money, would you just let him come and take whatever he wanted? I hope not! I hope you'd do whatever was necessary to protect your family and your belongings. That's what you have to do with cancer. Cancer comes like a thief and it tries to rob you of your health, your joy, and your relationships. Yes, you may be in for a struggle, and yes it could be painful, but you can beat the cancer and have a great life while you go through it! Your life is important and it's worth fighting for! You, my friend, were meant to be more than a survivor. You are a winner!

SHARE YOUR STORY

Now that I have shared my story
of hope and healing with you,
I invite you to share yours with me.

Each of us has a story to tell
and I would love to hear yours.

Please go to
www.sherryAsims.com
and click on
"Share Your Story"

ABOUT THE AUTHOR

Speaker and author Sherry Sims is more than a survivor, she's a fighter. In 1994, when faced with breast cancer, Sherry made a decision to not just *survive* the disease, but beat it; which she did. In the decades that followed, she has not only remained cancer free, but has devoted her life to encouraging others to fight and win.

In her recent memoir, *More Than a Survivor,* Sherry shares the inspiring true story of her struggle to stay positive and the miraculous outcome discovered under the surgeon's knife. Sherry's honest and often humorous portrayal of her fight delivers a powerful message of hope and healing.

Sherry has told her story on numerous television programs including *Make Your Day Count, Praise the Lord* and *Celebration!* She is also a popular speaker at conferences, churches, civic groups and breast cancer awareness events where she informs the public on cancer causes and cancer prevention strategies.

In addition to speaking, Sherry has extensive experience working behind the scenes for cancer charities. She has served as both board member and fundraising director for the Breast Cancer Assistance Program and is an active supporter of the American Cancer Society.

Sherry resides in the Tulsa, Oklahoma area with her husband, Randy, without whose support and encouragement this book would not have been possible.

To contact the author:

SHERRY A. SIMS
P.O. Box 330243
Tulsa, Oklahoma 74133-0243
www.sherryAsims.com